MW01287398

Without Mom,
With Spina Bifida

a memoir

by James Boucher

Copyright © 2017 by Rose Hall Media Company, LLP.

ALL RIGHTS RESERVED. No part of this book may be reproduced or transmitted in any form by any means, electronic or mechanical, including photocopying and recording, or by any information storage and retrieval systerm, except as may be expressly permitted by the 1976 Copyright Act or in writing from the publisher. Requests for permission should be addressed to: rightandpermissions@rosehallmedia.com

Library of Congress cataloging-in-publication data:

Boucher, James
Without Mom, With Spina Bifida / Rose Hall Media Company
cm
ISBN 978-1537191447

1. Boucher, James, 1975— 2. Family and Relationships 3. Birth defects—Spina bifida—Biography. 4. Disability services—Rhode Island.
Published by Rose Hall Media Company, St. Cloud, Minnesota

rosehallmedia.com

Rose Hall
Media Company

for Jarren Zucchi
(1983-2013)

Acknowledgements

This is the truth of my life as I remember it. All of the names have been changed to protect the privacy of people who didn't ask to be written about in a book.

I am grateful to my mother, who gave me life. I still miss her smiling face.

Thank you also to: my former home room teacher and friend; to M.C., who helped me to keep my sanity while I was in the hospital for six months; all the nurses and staff at Rhode Island Hospital for taking such great care of me; the people at Crotched Mountain Rehabilitation Center and School for taking care of me until I was old enough to go off on my own; and to K.L. who helped me at the beginning of my return to Rhode Island.

And a huge thank you to all the people at West Bay Residential Services who have taught me to trust, especially J.D. who has been like a father to me; J.P. and D.A, who have been like brothers to me; A.H., who helped me find my mom, and all of you who have become my family.

And thank you to Tracy Lee Karner for helping me find the best words to tell my story.

Chapter 1

THE SUMMER OF 1991, I WAS FIFTEEN AND desperately wanted to be stronger. I wanted to fight like a World Wrestling Federation Pro. I wanted to body slam the creep who dared to hurt my mother.

If I was a WWF fighter, I would kick Bill in the stomach and watch him double up on himself. When he fell forward I would push his head under my muscled-up legs, lean over his back and wrap my beefy arms around his stomach. Locking my fists together, I'd straighten up, lifting Bill like a five-pound sack of flour head down. I'd have him right where I wanted. I could break his neck just by sitting down fast.

But of course that wasn't going to happen. I had been born with Spina Bifada and knew I would never become an athlete. It was likely I'd never even get a driver's license. But I loved the raw body power of the World Wrestling Federation matches on television. I watched as often as I could. Sometimes I identified with the Babyfaces, the good guys: Hulk Hogan; Randy Savage; Lex Luger and the Texas Tornado.

The spectacular clashes between heroes and villains provided me with dramatic characters to cheer, jeer and imitate, depending on my mood. Sometimes when Bill pushed my mom around, or whenever he told her she should put me in an institution because I was feeble, I imagined him as one of the Wrestling Heels: Rick Rude; Sergeant Slaughter; Crush or Vader. *Thumbs down! Boo! You're a pig!*

I wanted to pulverize the SOB.

My t.v. heroes' bravery and resilience kept me going whenever I got scared, which was pretty often. I lived in a battle zone.

We lived in a blue-gray, three-story house in Woonsocket, Rhode Island, a historic New England mill town powered by the Blackstone River. There were six families in that house. We had half of the ground floor. A plywood ramp ran from the small, scruffy back yard up to the back door. It was my only way in and my only way out.

The kitchen is where I talked to Mom, because when I was in there, Bill wasn't. He wouldn't sit at the table with me. Bill was Mom's boyfriend at the time. I never knew my father. Mom said he left in 1975, shortly after I was born. Didn't want a disabled son. Sometimes I would ask about him, but I don't remember what she told me, if she told me anything interesting at all.

She worked at the jewelry counter in a department store. She was in her mid-thirties, tall, thin, and pretty. She had straight blond hair. She wasn't a perfect mother. She had a problem with alcohol and tended to get involved with men who mistreated her. But she was my mother. And I loved her. So when we were in the kitchen I tried to talk to her. I told her I was really uncomfortable with Bill, and with the life we were living. But being a teenager, I probably said something like, "I hate Bill. I hate the crummy life we're living."

The kitchen had a square wooden table that would seat four, but we never ate all together. Sometimes Mom could eat with me. Sometimes she'd eat with Bill. But mostly we all ate alone.

"What do you have against Bill?" Mom wanted to know.

Well, for starters, he hated me. He was an average-sized, Italian-looking guy with black hair and tan skin. He went out drinking a lot and came home intoxicated. He wanted me gone. Said I was a bad person who didn't belong in their home.

When he came home drunk, she decided to talk to

him about me.

Mom drank, too. I don't know how much, but her brain didn't work right. I mean, how dumb do you have to be, to attempt a conversation about your son's feelings with a drunk guy who hates your son and wants to put him in an institution?

Unsurprisingly, this encounter led to yelling, obscenities, hair-pulling, slaps and screams. That was Mom's normal pattern of interaction with the guys who lived with us.

Next, she would try to talk them into leaving. Her way of doing that was to yell and cry, saying, "Go! Leave me alone. Get out of here!"

Occasionally that would work and the guy would leave for a while, or forever. But usually her preferred method of de-escalating violence backfired. Things would get scarier. Eventually she would figure out the guy wasn't going to stop being violent and neither was he going to leave.

That's when she would leave. She'd be gone a few hours, or a few days.

And that's how I ended up on my own, hiding out in my room, hoping Bill was drunk enough to forget that their fight had been about me.

Chapter 2

AT THAT AGE, I WAS ALWAYS HUNGRY. BECAUSE Mom was gone, I was going to have to feed myself. So when Bill slept, or after he left, I would rummage around in kitchen looking for food. I might find a red and white can of chicken noodle soup, or maybe Chef Boyardee spaghetti. Now and then a t.v. dinner—frozen chicken with mashed potatoes and gravy. Mom bought the food I liked best, but she never bought much of it at once.

That previous January, Governor Bruce Sundlun had shut down forty-five banking institutions, freezing $1.7 billion worth of deposits. The Philadelphia Inquirer reported many businesses had laid off workers or closed. People who normally donated money to a Woonsocket soup kitchen called up to ask for food. Some people couldn't access savings funds to bury their recently deceased loved ones.

I wasn't aware of the community crisis surrounding me because it didn't change anything for my mother or me. We didn't have a savings account and frequently ran short of money to buy food. The important events most days, for most of my life, included getting myself into my wheel chair and rummaging through the cupboards for something to eat. It was normal not to find anything good in the cupboard or refrigerator.

I didn't know how long Mom would be gone and all I could think about was my stomach. There was a small Shaw's Market across the street behind our house and so I scrounged up 75 cents and wheeled myself over there.

I used to hang out with a bunch of older neighborhood tough guys. I just wanted to belong, and as long as I did what they wanted, they let me hang around them.

They wanted me to steal stuff for them. They taught me how.

First, I located an aisle with good stuff on a low shelf I could easily reach—cans of soup, beef stew, ravioli. Then I put the back of my chair between me and the camera and pulled up close to the shelf. Waited until no one else was in the aisle, slipped the goods into a backpack. Wheeled over to the candy aisle and repeated the procedure, loading up on Snickers, Milky Ways, and Hershey bars. Kept out a Reese's Peanut Butter cup, wheeled up to the check-out, and picked the cashier who looked most like a God-blesser—a person who automatically makes pathetic sad faces whenever she sees a kid in a wheel chair. Paid for one candy bar, then wheeled home.

I knew it was wrong. I had stopped hanging out with those guys who shoplifted for kicks. The last time I shoplifted to feed myself, I thought I would never do it again.

I like to believe I was developing a conscience, and wouldn't have stolen again even if I had been given the opportunity. But my life was about to change in a drastic way. I never shoplifted again, because that summer before I turned sixteen was the last time I ever had the opportunity to wheel myself over to Shaw's in Woonsocket.

In 1991, people didn't use the word *landline* because there was only one kind of telephone connection. Phones sat on tabletops or desks, or hung on the wall, immoveable. They had leash-like cords that tethered you to a specific spot. To talk to someone, you picked up a plastic barbell looking thing, held one end of it to your ear and the other to your mouth, and pushed buttons on a box to dial the number of the phone nearest the person you wanted to talk to. That meant you had to know where the person was. I couldn't call Mom because I didn't know where she was.

Mom couldn't call me from a car or from the bathroom at work because ordinary people didn't have cell phones back then. Maybe she could call from the grocery store, if she used a pay phone.

So I had to wait for her to call me. She wouldn't call as long as she thought Bill was in the apartment, so it might have been the next evening before I heard from her.

Ring-ring. The phone gave off a tinkly bell sound followed by a short pause. *Ring-ring.* If it was Mom, she would let it ring however long it took for me to get to the kitchen.

"Jamie!" Her smokey voice sounded relieved when I picked up. "Is Bill there?"

"No. When are you coming home?"

After she learned he was gone, she said she would meet me at the back door in five minutes, but she wouldn't be staying. I didn't ask why. I knew she was afraid Bill might hurt her.

Chapter 3

BECAUSE OF WHAT HAPPENED LATER THAT summer, all the details of that time are fuzzy in my mind. I remember she did not come into the house, but handed me a couple of bags of groceries. Rice Krispies and milk, frozen t.v. dinners, stuff I could make myself.

I can't say how long she was gone. Sometimes when she called, she would tell me she had left groceries in a bag by the back door. I should grab them before one of the neighbors found them. "And stay off your butt—take care of your bed sore or it's going to get worse."

I rarely left the house, but I also didn't stay off my butt. Sitting on my butt in my chair was the only way to get around, to get something to eat, to get to the living room to watch television.

The World Wrestling Federation stars were my best friends. Food was my second best friend. So I sat in front of the television, waiting, watching and eating—a chicken t.v. dinner with mashed potatoes and gravy, or a bowl of Cheerio's with plenty of sugar.

The Berserker is a wild-eyed guy with curly auburn hair, a full beard and mustache, and wearing a Norwegian Viking costume—shield, sword, horned helmet and brown leather tunic. He gestures like a caveman, holding his wrist and licking his hand while grunting, "Huss! Huss!" When he uses words, he shouts in a hoarse voice, as if a lifetime of constant screaming has damaged his vocal cords.

His manager Mr. Fuji wears a black tuxedo with pleated white shirt, a bow tie, and a bowler hat. He carries a cane and when the wrestlers get outside of the ring, the Berserker grabs Mr. Fuji's cane to whack his opponent, Greg Valentine.

Give me that cane, Mr. Fuji—let me whack Bill's head with it!

They tussle around for seven minutes until the Berserker wins the match by a count-out.

A lady with a blond poodle puff of hair on top of her head with matching poodle-hair ears down to her shoulders introduces the next match. "Weighing 255 pounds, Al Phillips!"

Phillips, bare chested, wearing a white shiny brief

and white shiny boots to contrast with his black shiny skin, marches around the wring with his arms above his head, pumping his fists.

Then the poodle-lady announces, "Colonel Moustafa!"

Moustafa goosesteps into the arena wearing a khaki soldiers uniform, beret, and a handlebar mustache. His boots have curly elf toes. His chest is decorated with medals. The announcers call him "a cruel vicious man...a pig!" The crowd gives him thumbs down. He hops into the ring and takes off his shirt to reveal a wrestler's suit. He looks Italian, like Bill.

Without waiting for the match to start, for no reason at all, Moustafa attacks Phillips and smacks his left collar bone, over and over, until Phillips collapses. He chokes him.

I feel like I can't breathe. *Get up Phillips!*

Phillips uses the ropes to struggle to his feet. Moustafa pulls him upright, shoves him across the ring into the opposing ropes. He ricochets back into the middle of the ring where Moustafa is waiting to clothesline him.

I hate that jerk!

Phillips flails, swings, misses. Moustafa throws him around like a sack of groceries.

This sucks! It's not fair!

Moustafa pounds his chest, spits on his hands, slicks the spit on his bald head and leans over Phillips to put him in a camel hold. He pulls back. Phillips is subdued. The bell rings and the match is over. But Moustafa is such a pig, he kicks Phillips a couple of times while he's down.

The crowd boos. *Thumbs down.* I boo. *I hate you, you jerk. I hate you!*

Whenever I heard Bill coming in, I knew he was bound to be drunk again. I would turn off the television, wheel myself to my room and turn out the lights, waiting for him to go away.

I can't remember whether Mom brought Pauline and Jack with her when she moved back in. I can't say for sure exactly when they showed up, but after they moved in with us, Bill was outnumbered.

Pauline had brown hair starting to gray and wore glasses. Jack was a medium-sized guy. Everyone in the house, except me, smoked.

Mom said they were going to help pay the rent. I wasn't quite sure how that was going to work, since they didn't have jobs, but they helped Mom take care of me, and for that reason I was glad they lived with us. I had people to talk to, people who stood up for me when Bill threatened to send me to an institution, people who made food for me, people who were always there and were pretty nice to me.

16

I wished that Pauline and Jack would live with Mom and me forever. But I knew something wasn't quite right. There were fights with Bill about them. They lived there, but they didn't pay any rent. Something had to give.

We humans all want the same thing—a home, a place where we feel connected by loving relationships. I got an inkling of what that feels like when Pauline and Jack lived with us. At the same time, I was terrified Bill would get his way and Pauline and Jack would have to leave. I knew it had to happen, but it was impossible for me to imagine the reason why Pauline and Jack would end up out of my life forever. I had no idea what happened next was even possible.

Chapter 4

IT WAS LATE AUGUST, 1991, AND I WAS IN THE living room watching television with Pauline and Jack. There was a knock on the door which we didn't answer, because Mom had told us not to open it for anyone.

Then came a loud crash, a splintering of wood, and the door flew off its hinges. The landlord stormed in. We were late with the rent, and the landlord had been calling her but she hadn't returned his calls. He looked around, cussed, and left.

We sighed with relief. Pauline and Jack did their best to close the door. Maybe one of them called Mom at work, but I don't know for sure. We went back to watching t.v., probably a game show like *The Price is Right*.

Mom was still at work when the landlord returned with EMT's and a social worker.

The EMT's measured my pulse, looked in my eyes, ears, throat, and pulled down my pants so they could check out my bedsore. They offered no explanations, small talk or apologies. They weren't exactly mean, but they sure were grim.

I had the feeling they didn't like what they were seeing. They wheeled me out, transferred me to an ambulance and took me to the emergency room of Rhode Island hospital in Providence.

The twenty minute ride was like being trapped in a bubble, with strangers peering in at me. If they talked to me, I barely heard them. All I heard were the thoughts deep inside of me, in that place where love and hope are connected to the only family you have ever known. I kept telling myself, "I wish my mom was here. I just wish she was here."

I continued thinking the same words at the hospital, where doctors and nurses, all strangers, hooked me up to an IV and then came and went, always in a rush, while they prepared a room in the hospital for me. Various people talked about what was in the drip—something to help my bedsore heal, something to rehydrate me. They wouldn't allow me to eat because they thought I might need surgery on the bed sore. But all of that sounded like radio static around the relentless echo in my head. *I wish Mom was here.*

I was admitted to the Potter Building, the old children's wing before Hasbro Children's Hospital was built in 1994. Day after day, nurses, doctors, and social workers came and went.

I wish I could remember the names and faces of all the people who were good to me. But everything about that time is blurry and all I remember is asking the friendliest of my caregivers, Paul, whether he had heard from my mom. When would she come?

Nobody had heard from her. She never came.

I lay there in my bed, on my right side or on my stomach so my bedsore could heal, feeling the starchy hospital sheets on my skin, staring at the sterile room, wondering what would happen to me. Trapped there, surrounded by the peculiar hospital smell of sickness, disinfectant, and helplessness, it was beginning to dawn on me that maybe my mother wasn't allowed to see me.

These strangers were taking better care of me than my mother had been able to, making sure I had nutritious food, dressing my wound, trying to keep my spirits up when too much anger or sadness seeped in and threatened to turn the world into a nightmare. Gradually I began to understand the truth. I missed my mom, but I didn't want to go back to that terrible situation.

But if I didn't go back, where would I go? A hospital is a transition place. If you don't die there—and clearly I wasn't going to die—you get well. You go home to your family. But suddenly I did not have a home, or a family.

Chapter 5

SPINA BIFIDA IS A DEVELOPMENTAL DEFECT. Mine was the most serious form—a myelomeningocele (pronounced my-e-lo-MENING-o-seal). Probably before my mom knew she was pregnant, part of my backbone, spinal cord and spinal canal did not fully close. This allowed a small membrane-covered sac to extend through the spinal opening, on the outside of my body. The sac contained spinal fluid, tissues that protect the spinal column, and portions of the cord and nerves.

Up to 90% of children born with a myelomeningocele also have a build up of fluid inside the skull (hydrocephalus). Within days of my birth, surgery repaired the spinal defect, but irreparable damage was already done. I get around with a wheelchair. Surgery was also necessary to install a ventriculo-peritoneal shunt in my brain, to help drain the extra fluid to my bladder. Without this shunt, fluid build up would cause me to suffer memory loss, disorientation and eventually death.

Doctors, hospitals and surgeries have been a normal part of my life. But this was the first time I was going through the health-care ordeal without my mom.

I also turned sixteen without her. I imagined the lives of other people who celebrated their sixteenth birthday. I pictured a young man finding a shiny black car in his driveway. Maybe he would be thinking about getting a job bagging groceries so he could pay for gas, or maybe his rich parents would just give him a credit card.

I pitied myself. I was officially on my own, frightened and confused.

I thought about my mom a lot. She was not a happy person, and I always wanted to make her feel better, make her smile. It was a terrible feeling, wanting to help her in some way, knowing that I couldn't, feeling like I had failed her.

She told me to stay off my bottom, and said my bed sore would get worse if I didn't listen. It was my own fault that I had to have surgery to repair my bed sore.

A parade of people came in and out of my room—tutors to help me with schoolwork, legal experts to help me figure out where and how to live the rest of my life. I would have to choose between foster care and an institution and they explained the advantages of each PT to me. Physical therapists were there to teach me how to be more self sufficient. Social workers wanted to help me deal with the anger, confusion, and feelings of abandonment. Often I felt on the verge of panic.

Paul became my favorite nurse. I pretended he was my big brother. While almost everyone was kind to me and took care of my needs, Paul gave me special treatment.

One night he came into my room, transferred me to a stretcher (I wasn't allowed to sit) and wheeled me out.

"Where are we going?"

"Guess!" He laughed and wheeled me into the elevator. He took me to the next building and when we arrived at the cafeteria, he treated me to a pizza. It was my last meal before my surgery, and he made sure I got my favorite food.

When I came back from the operating room after surgery, there was Paul. I learned later that he specifically asked to always be assigned to take care of me, just like a protective big brother would have done. And he would get me whatever I wanted to eat.

I wasn't used to being treated kindly.

Often when Paul said good morning, asked how I was doing, cared for my needs by giving me sponge baths, I was nasty. I wasn't a very good morning person. I didn't want to be woken up. I was away from home, there was nothing to worry about, my time should have been my own, and then people would come in and wake me. It really irritated me.

I would lash out, saying, "Leave me alone!" I didn't think I was being rude or mean, I just thought I was expressing my feelings. Even when I gave up on myself, I expected—I just assumed—my caregivers would not give up on me.

"Hey, man," Paul said. "You're not just expressing your feelings to an empty room. I'm here. I'm a *person*. See your roommates? They're not furniture; they're *people*. We have feelings, too. Your attitude affects us, and your attitude is not good."

All right! I knew what I ought to do, but often just couldn't be the person I wanted to be. Was I afraid? You bet I was. Disabled people are vulnerable and there's a long history of their exploitation. I wanted to be able to trust Paul, but honestly, I didn't trust anyone.

Paul wasn't the only person at Rhode Island Hospital who showed compassion and kindness to me. Jason was a patient in the room next to mine. I didn't ask what was going on with him or why he was there. I tended to keep to myself and think of only myself.

Jason's family was interested in how I was doing. The

hospital wasn't a very private place, and they overheard everything I was going through.

Jason was a bit older than me, but I didn't ask how old. I didn't know how to be interested in other people. I had always been kept away from other people, or I stayed away by choice.

Occasionally I would reach out to other kids at home, the neighbors, because I wanted them to know about my life, and that I was a decent person. But their mother wouldn't let them hang out with me. I assumed it was because I was different. But maybe it was because of my mother's reputation. In any case, outside of school, it was difficult to get anyone to talk to me or look at me.

I had never learned to ask the simple social questions— how are you, how old are you, why are you in the hospital?

I don't remember what Jason and his parents looked like, or what their voices were like, or anything specific about them or our conversations at all. I remember the hospital antiseptic smell, the noise, especially at night, how hard it was to sleep, people moaning in pain, sometimes yelling, monitor alarms going off at all hours, the nurses hurrying along the hallway. Mostly I remember my own physical and emotional pain.

When you're in a hospital alone, whenever you ask for anything, you have to wait, because there are other people who need something too. Sometimes you wait twenty minutes, which feels like a long time when you think your problem is urgent. When I was fifteen going on sixteen, being in the hospital was an endless excruciating experience.

Jason was brought up to believe in and respect God and Jesus. I knew this because I heard him talking to his family about their beliefs. No matter what he was going through, they would say, "Jesus will help you through it."

When Jason's parents weren't there, he would come in to my room to talk. I started to listen, mostly because I was bored with the usual sounds—television, monitor alarms, and people screaming—so I started tuning into his conversation with me. I also began eavesdropping more on his conversation with his parents.

After a while of listening, something inside of me wanted to learn what they meant when they said *Jesus will help you through it.* Although there were people talking to me, trying to keep my spirits up, I didn't really think they would help me through my problems. I thought only family could do that, and my family had disappeared from my life.

For a while, the staff in the hospital came to be like a family to me. At the same time, I knew they weren't in my life to stay. I couldn't emotionally attach to them because of that. I believed it was my destiny to be lonely for the rest of my life. How can a person by anything but lonely, without a real family?

I wanted to give up hope, but Jason gave me something to believe in. I asked him questions, and he and his parents began teaching me about Jesus.

That's when I began to believe that God is with me and always will be, whether I feel close to God or don't. Believing that God would take care of me satisfied my most critical need — for safety.

Jason and his family gave me a bible written for people who are just beginning to understand the Catholic faith. His parents put together a ceremony and gave it to me in my hospital room.

Jason gave me his phone number and told me to call whenever I felt lonely. I did call them for a while, but then somehow they slipped out of my life. I can't remember exactly how that happened.

Maybe it has happened to you too, that people you met, who were kind to you and changed your life in a small or big way, faded away like music posters stapled to telephone poles, exposed for months to the weather.

I developed a habit of letting people slip away, a habit that became hard to break and led to recurring loneliness. I couldn't quite believe the people I looked up to would want me around them.

Or maybe there was just so much else going on in my life that I wasn't capable of thinking about anything other than my problems. During my hospital stay I developed a latex allergy. Imagine a constant irritation that won't go away, no matter how you swat at it or scratch it.

And then they discovered I had sleep apnea. Sleep apnea means you're constantly on the verge of suffocation, you get no restful sleep, and you turn into a grinch who wants everyone to be as miserable as you are. And I was depressed, and I had an eating disorder, and my mom had abandoned me.

Yeah, I was a mess. I hate thinking of myself at that time. I felt like an utterly hopeless wreck of a human being, like a wrestler who had been beaten so bad, he'd never be allowed back in the ring.

I was aware that the Rhode Island Department of Children, Youth and Families was looking for a home for me. My mom either didn't want me or wasn't allowed to take me back. Whoever took me in would need to participate in and continue my treatment after I was discharged from the hospital.

All of my problems were written up in my medical charts and sent out to whomever would consider taking me in to care for me. I tried to comfort myself with dreams of being adopted into a happy family, but it didn't work. I had already turned cynical.

Without my mom, with spina bifida

Who in the world wants to care for a wheel-chair bound teenager with bedsores, with red, flaky, angry-looking skin, who snores and grouches, who is depressed, and who hoards and steals food and overeats? I was pretty sure I knew the answer to that question.

No one would want me.

Chapter 6

MY DCYF CASE WORKER WAS A MAN, AND unfortunately that's all I remember about him. I can't tell you whether he was old or young, tall or short, whether he was funny or had bad breath. That I paid almost no attention to him, tells you the depth of my self-concern during the approximately six months I was in the hospital. All the people around me seemed more like see-through ghosts than people.

One day my case worker brought a woman from Exeter, Rhode Island to my room. She was volunteering to take me into her home as a foster child. By then I already knew that going home to my mother wasn't an option. I had never heard of Exeter, and had no idea where it was. And strangely, I thought I wasn't interested in becoming part of a family.

Do you see what I was doing to myself? I was

miserable because I didn't have a family, and then, when I was offered a family situation, I decided I didn't want it. Because…. I don't know why I didn't want it.

The other option DCYF offered me was an institutional setting at Crotched Mountain in New Hampshire. (Crotch-ed is pronounced like bless-ed in older English, two syllables). I decided to go with that, thinking it would be better for me to get an education than to live with a family. Crotched Mountain had a special high school there. And intuitively I felt I would feel safe there. I told myself that getting a good education was better than being in a family.

It was fully my choice, but I couldn't shake the feeling that I was being pushed into moving out of state and away from my mother.

"It's your own decision, James," I kept telling myself, "no matter what anyone else thinks, you get to make this decision. It's entirely up to you to decide."

But instead of comforting me, the fact that it was up to me alone to determine my future scared the hell out of me. I felt powerless. My head buzzed and my stomach was queasy from constant worry.

In retrospect, I consider it a miracle that I had a choice. When I was sure nobody would want to help me, I was presented with two people/places who were willing to take me in. This is just one example of the many reasons I came to believe that God provides what I need.

So I signed medical release forms and filled out admission forms, and Rhode Island Hospital discharged me into the care of a man named Sam from Crotched Mountain. He was a nurse there.

He helped me pack my few clothes, my Bible from Jason's family, and a couple other gifts from nurses and people who knew I was entirely on my own. (I wish I could remember what those gifts were — but those bits of memory are entirely gone!)

It was Paul's day off, but he had heard I was leaving and came to say goodbye. I wish I had been mature enough to fully appreciate what that meant. He and my new nurse, Sam, wheeled me out into the hallway.

All the way to the elevator, the halls were lined with people—nurses, family members of other patients, and other staff, who had learned that I was moving to New Hampshire.

Hugs, handshakes, words of good luck and more than a few tears accompanied me down the hallway. I rode the elevator down with Sam and an orderly I didn't know, and exited the building to be wheeled out to the car. "Crotched Mountain" was written in bold letters on the vehicle. The logo included pine trees and a sunset, as if I was going on vacation to a luxury resort.

I looked back at the building I had called home for so many long months. Already all those farewell hugs, handshakes, good wishes and tears were drifting away, disappearing like wake behind a boat. Already in my memory, there was only a momentary trace of the first six months of the journey that took me away from Mom.

Goodbye Paul. Thanks for everything.

Right then, I made a silent promise to myself to try to be a better person. I wanted to make all that went wrong in my life, right. I wanted to leave behind all the emotional and physical wounds.

So, while Sam and the orderly transferred me to the back seat of the car, stowing my wheelchair and belongings, I said a silent goodbye to the painful past, and deluded myself into thinking that for the rest of my life, I would be in control, and I would make a good life for myself. The trunk slammed and shook the car.

The orderly ran back up the walkway. It was February, and bitter cold. Watching him dash into the warm building felt like watching my life—those fifteen years in Woonsocket, and the last six months in Rhode Island Hospital—run away from me.

And this stranger named Sam would drive me to a new home I had never seen, in a place I had never been and didn't know how to get to.

Chapter 7

SAM WALKED AROUND TO THE DRIVER'S SIDE of the car and opened the door. A rush of cold winter air filled the vehicle. He pulled his wool coat around his body while he positioned himself in the driver's seat, shivered, and turned the key. The car hummed while he let it idle to warm up. He fiddled with the heater, turned it to high, then turned to me and smiled.

"How are you doing back there?" he asked, trying to be friendly.

I didn't say anything, just nodded my head. I absolutely did not feel like talking to anyone.

So much for my resolve to always be a better person and think about other people's feelings.

Sam turned his attention to putting the car in gear, and pressed the accelerator. I paid particular attention to every detail. I was sixteen and badly wanted to drive, yet knew I never would.

I fixated on the driver and the vehicle. It was one way to not fret about my unknown future.

Driving is different in winter, I noticed. The air is frigid and the engine is sluggish, the ground is slick from pedestrian-packed snow. The wheels spin, throwing off wet snow and mud until they get a grip on the pavement and the car jolts forward. A strong wind might force you sideways until you hit a patch of salty slush. I paid attention to all that without it ever dawning on me that there are forces in the world that you really cannot control.

When I made up my mind to be a better person, I didn't think about the fact that I wouldn't be alone in the world. There would be other people in my new life, and I would have to learn to stop always thinking of myself as the most important person in the room. There would be forces of nature, and clocks and calendars—all sorts of frustrations to contend with. And I hadn't learned very much about how to manage frustration.

We were cruising north at 70 miles per hour. Sam drove and Sam talked. I sat in the back and brooded and tried to tune him out.

He was an older man, very friendly, with brown hair and glasses. I didn't make the effort to notice whether they were plastic or wire. He wanted to get to know me, he said.

I could tell he was trying to make me feel comfortable for the duration of the drive. It was nice of him to attempt to make me feel less anxious about moving away from the only life I had ever known. But he talked so much that I kind of wanted him to shut up and leave me alone to think. He wouldn't shut up, so I decided to start answering some of his questions, to give my ears a break from his voice.

"Why are you moving?" he asked.

"Umm. I don't have a family. I'm going to school in New Hampshire."

"What are you looking for in your new life?"

Why should I open up to this guy? I asked myself. I'm never going to see him again. I gave him the shortest answer possible, probably something like, "I'm going to get my high school diploma."

"What are you interested in?"

I already had figured out from my time in the hospital that getting attached to this guy was not worth my effort. No matter how nice he was, one of us was going to move on at some point, and I'd never see him again. Caregivers might be wonderful while they're working with you, but my cynicism never failed to remind me that they're paid to be good to you. When their job with you is over, they're not going to be coming around to hang out, I told myself. They have their own lives, their own family and friends. I'm just their job.

I told myself I was just being realistic. Sam had no real connection to me that would keep him in my life. He wasn't my father, my uncle, or my brother. He could never be a substitute for family.

But his question was still hanging there—*what do you like to do?*

"I like to watch WWF wrestling on television," I told him.

Even giving him that much felt like I was being violated somehow, like he didn't have a right to any part of me. But I was trying to be polite, and also trying to shut him up so I could sit quietly, thinking my own thoughts.

It was a long drive, and I was short in the willpower department. So eventually his genuine interest in me won me over a little bit. I started listening when he explained about my new room and the people I might meet. He said he would make sure to help me get my medications ordered, get the distribution squared away so there would be no interruptions to my care.

And a few hours later, we approached the bottom of Crotched Mountain, which was, in fact, a real snow-and-ice covered mountain like nothing I'd ever seen before. It looked dangerous. I didn't know how we were going to make it up the steep driveway, but we did.

Sam helped me get out of the car, carried my stuff to my room in the medical wing, and made sure I felt comfortable. He really was a nice guy. He didn't abandon me, but stuck around for an hour or two, making sure the nurses understood my medications.

"See you around," he said when he left.

"Yeah," I thought. "Probably not."

I had developed the expectation that people would walk out of my life and never come back.

Chapter 8

MY RHODE ISLAND LIFE WAS CITY HUSTLE-BUSTLE
and crowds of recognizable people. The only landscape
I had ever known was flat, made up of asphalt, concrete,
and 19th Century houses. Mills and factories surround
industrial rivers and the industrialized Narragansett Bay,
as if to subdue nature for strictly commercial use.

In contrast, New Hampshire was quiet, a view of hills
and valleys, and fresh mountain air. Nature was free to
be itself, sometimes beautiful and breathtaking, often,
especially in winter, terrifyingly harsh.

I thought I was allergic to smog. It turns out I was
allergic to trees, grass and flowers. My allergies went
wild in New Hampshire. And although there were fewer
people, every single one of them was a complete stranger.

And I had a roommate to get along with.

The rooms were like hospital rooms, with two beds

per room. We each had a dresser for our clothes, and a sink to share. The communal bathrooms (one for men; one for women) were down the hall. The walls were painted blueish gray, the floors were white tile. Very antiseptic, but keep in mind this was a medical rehab center, not a house. My bed was near the door. My roommate's empty bed was near the window with a view of a courtyard with snow and trees. It was getting dark, almost dinner time. Sam asked if I wanted help unpacking, but I wanted to do it alone.

I was supposed to supply my own bed linens, but I had none. I had almost nothing. All I owned were the things people gave me while I was in the hospital—my Bible, a few clothes, some little gifts. Rhode Island Hospital had given me sheets to take along.

In the twenty minutes it took me to unpack, I wondered what my roommate would be like, and who I would meet at dinner.

People stopped by periodically to ask if I needed anything. I was aware they were trying to make me feel comfortable, but I was reluctant to ask for anything. My closest companion in those days was a negative feeling of mistrust.

My major concern was getting comfortable in my own skin, being on my own in a setting of strangers, getting to know my cohorts—adults and teenagers who needed medical rehab for disabilities, injuries, and brain trauma. I would also need to get to know the staff.

Dinner was at 5:30 and I wheeled myself to the cafeteria. I was hungry, because I hadn't eaten since lunch. A staff member told me to sit wherever I wanted to. So I chose the first available place closest to the door, in case of an emergency. I am always thinking about safety, and getting out of a room in case of flood or fire.

There were long tables, each seating six or eight people. And there were big bay windows with a view of the mountains to the east. Later, I would come to this room early in the morning to watch the pink and yellow sunrise.

I don't remember who was at my table that night. I knew I ought to try to make friends, but the only thing on my mind was myself—whether my bed sore would ever heal, whether I would be able to do my schoolwork while being mostly limited to bedrest, whether I would ever feel comfortable.

I hardly spoke to anyone, and would like to say I listened, but really, I wasn't listening. I hadn't yet learned how.

The food came in from a food service company, all prepared and dished up on trays that staff pulled out of a unit. Of all the meals I ate there, none stands out as being particularly good or bad, or memorable. When I was home in Rhode Island, I often thought about food. But food wasn't very much on my mind during my years at Crotched Mountain. I finally had more important things to think about, like my future and what I might do with it.

After dinner, some people went to the community room to watch television, but I wanted to get settled and went back to my room. My roommate was there getting ready for bed with staff assistance. He was in a wheelchair, like me, and using an eye-gaze board with letters on it. This told me he was nonverbal. It was my first experience with someone who couldn't speak.

"Great," I thought. "I get a roommate who can't communicate with me. If this doesn't work out, it certainly won't be my fault."

But the staff person who was helping him, also helped us communicate.

"Hi," I said. "My name is James."

My roommate wore glasses and had a head stick. A head stick is like a helmut with a stick attached to it—and he used the stick to point to things he wanted, or to a specific letter on his board. He pointed to his letter board, directing me to pay attention.

J - A- C-K, he spelled.

"Hi, Jack," I said. "I guess we're going to be

roommates."

I told him my story—most of what you've read so far, and then began asking him questions. "Why are you here?"

It was a slow process, but letter by letter and with help from the staff person, who spent about an hour helping us get to know each other, I learned that he needed a lot of personal assistance and was learning how to communicate better. His goal was to learn to be a little more independent.

"My goal is to get over my bed sore and get my high school diploma."

I probably wasn't very friendly to him, because my interest in him was mostly curiosity—I thought his method of communication was fascinating.

That he was able to communicate at all blew me away. Still, in typical fashion I was thinking more about myself than about him. It looked to me like communicating with Jack was going to be a continual game of twenty questions. Whenever he looked toward the hallway, was I going to have to guess: *do you want the door closed? or the lights off?*

After the business of getting to know my roommate, I went to talk to the nurse about my medical needs, settled into bed, and tried to prepare myself mentally for the next day. I would have to learn to communicate my needs and try to find my way around the campus, which, from

47

my wheelchair perspective was many long hallways, a lot of hills.

Chapter 9

MY FIRST MORNING ON THE MOUNTAIN I WOKE up on my own in Lower Mellon, a hospital rehabilitation unit, with the sensation of starting an exciting new chapter in a book. But, not knowing what to expect also gave me an uncomfortably shaky feeling, as if something dangerous was always about to happen.

What I didn't know when I arrived, and was too young to appreciate while I was there, is that Crotched Mountain was founded in 1953 as a nonprofit, charitable organization that serves the needs of children and adults with disabilities, and their families. With a campus of 1,400 acres, with a school, hospital, outpatient clinic, aquatic center, residences, athletic complex and the nation's longest accessible trails, it really is something like the luxury resort I imagined when I saw the sunset and pine trees logo on the car that brought me there.

I got special treatment there. But I was stuck in that place of victimization, in which I thought I deserved special treatment. At the time, I didn't fully appreciate all they did for me. They renewed my hope and restored my life. Today I'm very grateful for that.

But I won't beat myself up for being an imperfect teenager. I'm not the only human who has missed being grateful for blessings at the moment of experiencing them.

My roommate Jack was already gone by the time I woke up that first morning. I've been able to get up on my own since I was three or four, mostly because I had to learn how to get out of bed, or I would have been left there most of the day and night.

Staff helped me work the showers in the communal bathroom. I dressed myself, went to the cafeteria for breakfast, and prepared for school. I took the elevator down to the ground floor with other students, none of whom I yet knew, and followed the flow of people walking, people wheeling, and people leaning on walkers through a long tunnel to the school building to my homeroom.

I had been given my homeroom teacher's name, Dee C., and asked someone where her room was.

"Four doors down," he said.

None of the rooms were numbered, so I counted the

doorways and stopped at the fourth. "Is this Mrs. C's room?"

"Yes. I'm Dee." I wasn't aware that students called their teachers by their first names. That was awkward for me. It seemed slightly disrespectful. Was that a New Hampshire thing? Or just a Crotched Mountain thing?

It was an interesting way to form a teacher-student relationship. It made clear that the teachers were trying to make us feel comfortable. And it gave me the immediate sense I was going to have some control over my education and my choices.

Dee came over to talk to me, to reassure me that it was okay to come in. She directed me to my desk and introduced me to the rest of the class. "Class, I'd like you to welcome James Boucher."

Those who were able to, stood while the whole class said in unison, in friendly voices, "Hi, James." Evidently they had rehearsed this. It made me feel immediately welcomed and respected, and started the long, slow process of chipping away at my mistrust and cynicism.

Dee was average height, wore glasses and had really short, black-brown, straight hair. She was wearing a dress and appeared to be in her late thirties or early forties. Her voice was soft, hard to hear if you were in the back of the room, I imagine, but I was in the middle of the room. I enjoyed listening to her talk, even when she was only going over all the rules and regulations.

If I had been more open to relationships, I might have developed a crush on her. She was so kind and helpful. But I never thought of her, or of anyone else, as a potential "relationship" in those days. I was only concerned with surviving.

The doctor's office was near my room, and after classes I went in for my first appointment, a check up. They told me I needed a flu shot and I told them I already had gotten one. But it wasn't recorded in my file, and so, officially, I still needed a flu shot. The second dose gave me the flu—or at least that's what I was convinced of at the time. A few hours after the shot, the aches and pains, fever and chills of flu had me in their grip so tight I could barely wheel myself to my room. I spent the next few days in bed.

Today I realize that it's entirely possible that the reason Rhode Island hadn't recorded the vaccine is because I hadn't received one. I was sixteen, stressed out and frightened, and not all of my perceptions were accurate. And it's not likely the vaccine "gave me" the flu. Probably I had been exposed to it and coincidentally was coming down with it before I got the vaccine. Maybe the shot protected me from having a worse case.

But at that point in my life, I needed to find someone

or something to blame for all my huge problems. At that point in my life, I was absolutely convinced that someone holding a hypodermic filled with vaccination, was the cause of all my unhappiness.

Caregivers kept coming into my room to nurse me, to keep me hydrated, giving me medication I didn't want. I was frustrated and angry. I wanted to get out of bed and get on with my life. I was angry at whoever was supposed to have recorded the shot I thought I had been given in Rhode Island, a vague rage that I took out on my caregivers, who were annoying me to smithereens. I wanted to go to school, and if I couldn't go to school, I just wanted to be left alone. I was obnoxiously rude.

It felt like I was in bed for half a lifetime, but it was only a few days, which I mostly slept through. Whenever I was awake during that time I obsessed on the problems I was going to face when I was well enough to get up.

I was going to have an uphill battle to establish myself as a person other people would want to be around.

I felt like some ogre had taken over my body and was making me act like a jerk. I knew I wasn't behaving like the good person I had promised to be, and I didn't understand why Jesus hadn't magically transformed me into a saint. I felt betrayed by that, too. I had expected miracles.

For reasons I don't know, my caregivers understood.

I've come to see that most people who get into the caregiving profession have natural empathy. They're able to put themselves in someone else's place and imagine what it's like to be someone who is having a hard time. It would be a long time before I learned that I ought to try to do that, too.

Chapter 10

FINALLY I WAS ABLE TO START MY REGULAR routine of going to school. My favorite class was science, because I liked the teacher, Jenny, and I liked the subject matter. I also like that the class was sometimes one-on-one. At the most I worked with two other students. I liked that kind of special attention.

Jenny was tall and had long brown hair. Wore glasses. When she taught, she was by-the-book strict. She was easy to get along with, as long as I did what she wanted.

One day, she put a dead frog on a tray and asked me to cut into it and look for its heart, lungs, and liver. The smell was overwhelmingly bad. And I just couldn't bring myself to cut into something that was once living. So I sat there and stared at it, afraid to touch the scalpel because I was sure I'd cut myself. I told Jenny I didn't feel comfortable. I didn't want to dissect that frog.

"Not doing it will affect your grade," she said.

"What do you mean?" I wanted to know. I wanted to stay on track with my grades so I could graduate. I didn't have a lot of leeway, as my long history of frequent absences from school in Woonsocket had made me a pretty poor student. I was determined to change that. "I want to do good in this class. I want to graduate."

"Then you'll just have to do this project," she said in the kindest possible way.

So I picked up the scalpel and forced myself to make the first cut. I had terrifying images of the scalpel developing a mind of its own and turning on me, puncturing my lung, cutting out my tongue. Or maybe the scalpel would hack the frog to pieces like a crime scene. And then my worst nightmare would happen, I'd get sent to the principal's office.

I had no idea what would happen, but the threat—*you'll be sent to the principle's office*—conjured up a black hole of danger-danger-danger! A state of nothingness, an invalidation of my existence as a decent human being.

So I cut the frog—one tentative little slit in the abdomen. And then I quietly freaked out.

Jenny saw the look on my face—utter disgust—and didn't say anything. I don't think she wanted to embarrass me in front of my classmates. She just waited. And so I made another cut. *Ugh. The tiny heart.* Cut. *The itty-bitty lungs.* Cut. *The pathetic liver.*

After class Jenny told me I would never have to do that again. "You weren't looking very well," she said. "But you got through it, and it's the only dissection we'll be doing."

Whew! Well at least I'll never have to do that again.

I hated the trips back to Rhode Island for doctoring. As a sixteen year old, I just didn't understand the intricacies of insurance regulations, and the bureaucratic business of institutions. And frankly it pissed me off.

But meanwhile I kept experiencing good things at Crotched Mountain, and opportunities to grow. Jenny helped us make a pinhole projector to watch a solar eclipse. And my life in rehab at Lower Mellon at Crotched Mountain passed quickly, mostly pleasantly. I had caring people who advised and helped me, I had plenty to do, and I was given opportunities to participate in activities that I had never even dreamed of.

Although I would never become a World Wrestling Federation superstar, I actually became an athlete, as a twenty-five meter freestyle swimmer, competing in the Special Olympics at the University of New Hampshire. I can't remember what my place was, but I didn't lose, and I felt good about that. I swam hard because the pool was brutally cold and I, wearing a lifejacket, swam as fast as

I could to get to the finish line. I had one goal, which my body worked hard to accomplish for me. *Get your butt out of this water before you freeze to death!*

I also became a Student Council member and was eventually elected president by my peers. I campaigned with integrity and honesty, and stood by my promises. My first months at Crotched Mountain became a time of innocence and happiness for me.

And then I took a major step toward adulthood, and that complicated everything.

Chapter 11

I MOVED OUT OF THE HIGHLY-SUPERVISED communal residence, shared with thirty-to-forty other people, and into the apartment program, with all its privileges and opportunities to make immature choices. At first, I was high on the privileges and didn't understand the responsibilities that are inherent in privilege. I felt so very grown up. I believed I was ready for a relationship.

Bella was "with" someone else when I met her. She was the girlfriend of my new roommate, Bryce. It was clear to me she wasn't happy with him.

She was in a wheelchair like me. She was short and heavy-set with short, straight blond hair with bangs. No glasses. I don't remember what color her eyes were.

Actually, I didn't really look at her much. I listened, rather than looked. Her voice was interesting. The pitch and volume of her voice went up and down, depending on her mood. Most of the time, when she was talking to me, her voice was gentle and pretty. But if she got angry, she got loud and a little screechy. I liked listening to her.

I could see that Bryce wasn't treating her well. And right under his nose, I started caring for her. Of course he was threatened by me, and that caused some tension in our room. But pretty soon we talked honestly, and I told him that I didn't think he was treating her well—trying to control her and keep her away from other people, making her sit by him when she wanted to sit by other people. I intended to be her friend and treat her better than he did.

I have to admit that we wouldn't have been able to work all that out on our own. We had professional support at every corner, people who guided us into communicating and treating each other with respect.

Bella and I really liked each other, but we were very young, and we fell into a relationship fast. For her, I was the way out, the escape from Bryce. For me, she was a possibility to have a family, to stop feeling abandoned.

We got close too quickly, and talked about plans for being more than just a couple. We thought we would get married. Her mother kept reminding her that she was too young.

I didn't have a mom to advise me. Crotched Mountain had rules that kept us safe. Of course I was too young to know who I should spend the rest of my life married to, but I didn't want to believe that.

When Bella graduated and moved out of Crotched Mountain, we officially ended our relationship. I tried to reach out to her once, about a year after, but she seemed perfectly happy without me, so I let it go.

That's the sanitized version of the Bella story, and it's true. That's what happened. The sanitized version is the way I remember the story today—a good story about growing through disappointment into maturity. It was part my slow acquisition of understanding, acceptance, and hopefully forgiveness for myself as well as for the people I felt hurt by.

Now let me give you a short description of what it felt like to learn those lessons of finding and losing my first love. There were tender bruises on my heart and lungs. Confusion kept a tight-chested vice-like grip on my thoughts, my emotions, my desires, and my needs. It was an emotionally violent way to learn about letting go.

You know what I mean. You've suffered your own heartbreak, haven't you?

I had a lot going on during the time I thought I was in love with Bella. Along with having severe physical limitation and medical problems, I felt all alone in the world — cut off from every family member I had ever known. I was trying to figure out how I was going to finish school, and wondered what the rest of my life would look like. I looked at the future through a very focused lens.

I mostly thought about getting back to Rhode Island to find my mom. This might be when I started planning on becoming a teacher. I had a fantasy that I could become a teacher like Dee and Jenny, help kids with disabilities, and at the same time earn enough money to be independent, make my own decisions, and make a home for my mom and me.

If I were a teacher, I'd have money to pay for a house and groceries. And my mom wouldn't have to rely on drunk, abusive boyfriends to help support her.

Chapter 12

IN 1996, I WAS ABOUT TO TURN TWENTY-ONE. I decided I was ready to leave Crotched Mountain. I wanted to go back to Rhode Island, to reconnect with my mom and my remaining family members, my aunt and her children, my cousins.

My relationship with my cousins was nothing but a fantasy. The three of them were small children, the youngest was an infant. I imagined that they would want a relationship with me just because we were blood relatives. They didn't even know me.

I had case workers in both Rhode Island and New Hampshire, and my Rhode Island case worker recommended West Bay Residential Services as the best place for me, but he wanted me to be part of the decision-making process. He was going to bring people up from Rhode Island for a lunch meeting.

Crotched Mountain provided a special meal, with turkey, ham, roast beef, and egg salad finger sandwiches, and we could choose our condiments—mustard or mayo. We had salad, soda, coffee, and choices of cookies like chocolate chip and oatmeal raisin. I'm not sure if it was the food or the reason we were meeting, but it is the most memorable meal I had while I was in New Hampshire. I wanted to load up my plate.

I behaved myself and didn't go overboard. I wanted to make a good impression.

Executive Director Ted was a short, stocky Rhode Island Italian. He wore glasses, wore a dressy-casual shirt., and probably khakis. He and I had an immediate connection. He seemed to understand where I was coming from, and I told myself, "Hey, I can trust this guy."

In order to move on with my life, I knew I needed to start trusting people. I was already twenty-one and had no real plan for myself. I needed people to guide me.

Nurse Ellen was a tall, dark-haired, soft-spoken woman. She wasn't wearing nurses' scrubs, just regular casual clothes. She gave me the idea that she wasn't going to pull any punches. I was going to have to do what she expected of me, or we wouldn't get along very well. That also gave me a sense of trust, because I was going to be around people who cared about my well being.

Maggie was an Assistant Director for West Bay. After

I moved to West Bay, she was always very sensitive to my needs and the needs of people I lived with, asking questions to make sure we were comfortable and happy. I liked her right away, too.

So, surrounded by people I felt safe with, I decided to move to Rhode Island, into one of the houses of West Bay Residential Services. They were remodeling a house, which I would share with three roommates.

Ted called me periodically to keep me updated on the construction process. They were making it wheelchair accessible on the inside, which meant larger doorways, completely remodeling the bathrooms, and arranging the kitchen so that we could access the sink and necessary items from the lower cabinets—silverware, pots and pans.

Finally I settled into my new home in Rhode Island, with my three roommates, all women. Life at home worked out pretty well. I found it easy to to be the only guy. The staff and I worked on getting to know and understand each other.

I went to Meeting Street Center, an agency in Providence that works to bring out the best in young people of all abilities. They helped me try out jobs to find my aptitudes and preferences.

I was involved with People in Partnerships, a social

services agency that helped me learn basic computer skills, (typing drills to get my speed up, learning to use Microsoft Word) and gave me training in a hospital cafe.

I hadn't yet caught on to the fact that no one was suggesting I become a teacher. I thought they were training me for preliminary jobs, the ones that would get me through college. I believed I was going to earn a professional salary, buy my own house, and move my mom in with me.

I was answering phones for West Bay, and enjoying my new job there when I was called into the office. I was failing to get messages to people, failing to connect calls—and this had been happening for some time. I wasn't capable of handling that much of a job, and they needed to find something more appropriate for me to do.

My next job involved putting packets together and answering the phone for just one person, Myla. I could manage that without messing up. My next job—sorting piles of invoices and papers for Hasbro toy company. Boring work, which I didn't feel was right for me.

I wanted to be a disc jockey. I wanted to express myself. I wanted to do something that matters.

And then I heard about a group called Very Special Arts of RI, a statewide organization that provides programs and opportunities for people with special needs. I began writing. Eventually I wrote a poem.

I Put Pen to Paper

When I put pen to paper
I feel a surge of energy flow within me
and down to the paper
forming into words.

Emotions and thoughts flood my mind,
spinning, rolling like a tornado
spreading its wrath across the face of the page.
When I put pen to paper

I take a deep, slow breath,
relaxing my arm, hand and mind.
I let go of the sounds around me,
focusing only on myself.

When I put pen to paper
I feel that nothing in the world can break me
away from all my thoughts, feelings
and the words that make all these poems flow.

When I put pen to paper I'm free.

I discovered that I enjoyed creative expression. Doors were being opened for me that I never even knew existed. My poem won the 1996 Ginsberg Prize, and I was honored at an awards ceremony in downtown Providence. *The Providence Journal* wrote an article about me. I was on my way to the top of the world.

And then reality came crashing in again.

Chapter 13

THE REALITY OF MY LIFE IS THAT I HAVE SERIOUS medical problems. After I won the Ginsberg award, I underwent a major surgery that would allow me to catheterize myself through my bellow button. It worked for a few months, but then failed.

The second surgery placed a small hole in the side of my bladder, with a catheter connected to a leg bag and at night, an overnight bag. This involves a trip to the hospital every six weeks or so for maintenance.

I spent a lot of time in the hospital during the years I chased my dream of becoming a teacher and reuniting with my mother.

I enrolled in a computer class at the Community College of Rhode Island (CCRI), and I volunteered as a mentor for a young man with special needs.

Tim was thirteen, short and stocky, not in a chair but

walked with a limp. I don't remember much about the way he looked. Getting along with him wasn't difficult. He was smart, funny, interesting. I wouldn't have agreed to work with someone who was looking to give me a hard time. I helped him with basic computer skills, to make him feel comfortable around computers, typing, searching the internet, reading the screen.

We met through a program called Advocates in Action at a workshop at the Comfort Inn in Pawtucket. After we had spend a couple of sessions together, he had a special request.

He said, "I want my friends to join us."

His friends were participating in the workshop, too, working one to one with mentors, but they wanted to make it a group thing.

Being in a group helped Tom focus. He stopped looking around the room, trying to see what everyone else was doing.

When I was given full control over the group. I felt like a real teacher. Cool!

I had material from Advocacy in Action, to teach my students about civics and how government works, how to read directions, how to work in a team, how to be a leader.

They also had their own work to focus on. I was supposed to be their mentor, directing their attention to the tasks and keeping them focused, assisting them with their homework, and answering questions. Their job was to do the work.

It wasn't long before sessions got out of hand. They were young. They didn't understand the importance of what they were doing, and weren't interested in learning. They got distracted by other things going on around them. It wasn't that they were intentionally bad, they were just young teenage boys.

"This is going to be fun, but structured," I told them.

I had to use my big voice—to bring them back to attention when they weren't paying attention. It was a struggle for me, being in the teacher role. I didn't like having to ask them to focus. I hated being a teacher.

I had to report back to the people who were above me, and told them it wasn't working. I was growing frustrated. The boys weren't focused, they didn't care about what we were asking them to learn. I liked them, but I didn't like that they didn't care to learn. It felt like they were purposely undermining me, thwarting my goal to teach them.

After school was out for the summer, I never went back.

I had failed with the students and with my goal to become a teacher. Was I defeated because I was trying to teach the way I was taught, and didn't have any other methods to draw from? Was I defeated because it just wasn't working to my satisfaction and I have no tolerance for people who don't try to learn? In any case, I stopped. I gave up on my goal.

At first it wasn't hard to accept that I wasn't going to be able to support myself by becoming a teacher. I had won a poetry award, and while I was doing all this school work with the kids, I was still writing poetry.

Aha, I decided, *I will be a professional poet.*

I submitted poems to places that were poetry oriented. One place contacted me and said that if I gave them $7,000 they would publish my book. I felt terrible that I didn't have the money.

No one told me, or if they told me I wasn't listening, that poetry and money don't exist in the same planes of reality. Poetry is meaningful and important, but it's like breathing. Most people don't get paid to breathe. Even the most successful professional poets have to support themselves with other careers—teaching, selling insurance, waiting tables, being lawyers, designing landscape projects.

But I didn't know that, and thought that because I wasn't getting paid to publish, I was a failure. I asked myself what I was supposed to do with all the words in my head, the words I wanted to share with people.

The fact that I had no answers to that question put me in a funk of regret and misery. I would never be able to share my thoughts with anyone. No one would ever understand me.

Chapter 14

MY WILL TO SURVIVE FORCED ME TO come up with a reason to live.

Maybe I couldn't support myself or support my mom, but I could still reconnect with my mom. After all, I was an adult, twenty nine years old, and DCYF had nothing to say anymore about my relationship with her.

My West Bay team was eager to help me. In 2004 they helped me locate my aunt Karen, Mom's sister. She had been trying to distance herself from Mom because they had entirely incompatible lifestyles and values.

Karen was living in northwestern Rhode Island, in the apple orchard part of the state. I phoned her.

"It's time for me to be in touch with my mom. Can you help me?

Long hesitation, "Um. I don't know."

It was obvious she didn't want to get involved. Or

maybe she didn't want me to get involved with my mother again, to go through what I had been through as a child.

She talked about family memories, she mentioned her three children, my cousins. She said that her grandparents came from Poland. She said somebody went to college, somebody else passed on.

Was she trying to get me to forget that I had asked specifically about my mom?

I asked her again, "Can you help me make contact with Mom?"

She reluctantly gave me a phone number and address. Mom was still living in Woonsocket.

I dialed the number. The phone rang. Butterflies in my stomach.

"Hello?" Of course she didn't have caller ID. Of course she wasn't expecting to hear her son's voice on the end of the line.

"Is this Gayle?"

"Yes. Who is this?"

"Mom, this is Jamie." I used my birth name.

I had changed my name to James because I disliked hearing myself called Jamie, but she knew me as Jamie. Just saying the name was like speaking a curse.

Jamie was who she yelled at when she was drunk and

angry. Jamie was who she and her boyfriends argued about.

Silence. Then it hit her. *Jamie!*

Small talk. Time passing. Keeping my goal in mind, but not mentioning that I wanted to see her again.

I wasn't sure whether she could get in trouble for contacting me, but I knew she couldn't get in trouble if I initiated the contact, so I called her again. The second conversation was a little warmer. The third one even better.

So I asked her the big question.

Do you want to meet?

We arranged a reunion, dinner in Woonsocket at Burger King.

I was in the van with my driver. Angie, one of my residential directors, drove her own car. She went along to support me, and to ensure my safety. We didn't know what to expect, we were blindly going into new territory.

When we got to Burger King, Mom was waiting at the front door of the restaurant, smiling. She looked the same. She hadn't changed in thirteen years.

We went in, found our table, ordered.

Small talk.

Then I mustered up the courage to show her the gift. I hadn't been able to give her anything in thirteen years, so I made her a ceramic lion. I painted the colors by looking at a book. I was very proud of it—it looked fairly professional.

She said she was proud of me, how I had grown, who I had become. She opened her arms and hugged me, and said she wanted to see me again.

"I'll call you," I told her. She was okay with that.

Our second meeting was at a sit-down Chinese restaurant in Woonsocket. We hadn't told Mom where I was living. This was a precaution against her showing up, unannounced. The same travel arrangements were made and soon my driver and I were in the van again, Angie following in her car.

This time Mom wasn't waiting at the door. We waited outside in our vehicles, but didn't see her. My driver went inside to look for her, but there was no one inside who looked like her. We waited twenty minutes.

Mom didn't show up.

The drive home was like the silence of four a.m., when you can't sleep and don't want to get out of bed to face your lonely self in the dark.

I don't remember how it happened, when or where,

but I must have seen her again because she introduced me to a man who wasn't at Burger King when we met the first time. Doug was her boyfriend. He was medium build and had glasses. I couldn't get any sense of what kind of man he was, whether he treated Mom better than her other boyfriends, or treated her badly. She told me there were good and bad times with him.

I dared to believe again in our future, a time when Mom and I would be together in safety, just being together like a mother and son should.

On May 1st, 2005, Aunt Karen called me at home.

"You won't believe this.

"Won't believe what?"

She took a deep breath.

"What?" I asked.

"Your mom passed unexpectedly."

I didn't know how to deal with news like that so I shut down. I felt nothing. I saw nothing, said nothing, heard nothing, thought nothing—as if I was with Mom.

I felt dead.

Chapter 15

Strangely, life went on. All the daily stuff—the sun rising and setting as a signal to get up, eat, work, go to bed and get up again—it all just kept happening.

We have psychologists on the team at West Bay Residential Services. I am cared for by an agency of good people who won't let me stay in a shut down state of mind. So with much help I began to do that "working through it," thing.

My aunt Karen came to my house to tell me about my mom's will.

Mom wanted to be cremated. Karen asked me to sign papers to allow them to turn Mom into ashes. I didn't want it to be that way, but I decided to give Mom what she wanted.

After her cremation, because I was the next of kin,

my staff took me to retrieve her remains. We drove to the funeral home about half an hour away. I couldn't tell you where it was or what the name was. I was in a fog that didn't allow me to see details.

"I'll come in with you so you don't have to do this alone," my staff said.

Riding home with mom's remains in the van felt eerie. I kept her remains for a week while I planned the release of them over the water, where she wanted. It gave me a chance to say goodbye.

I called Mom's sister Karen and Mom's boyfriend Doug. We all agreed to meet at Galilee on Point Judith, Rhode Island near George's restaurant. That's where Mom wanted to be.

Galilee is a fishing village, named for the Biblical Galilee, the home of four fishermen—Peter, Andrew, James and John—who were disciples of Jesus. It's a pretty little place, a favorite of many Rhode Islanders.

I never learned why it was significant to Mom. There is so much about her I never knew, never will know.

We met early morning in late May. It was cold on the water. Blue-gray sky, a storm rolling in. Waves weren't too high yet. Karen was there with her husband, and her three children, my cousins. For twenty minutes we waited for Doug. It was getting colder, windier, and later.

Karen sprinkled Mom's ashes into the water and we said goodbye.

A while later, we held a memorial service for Mom at West Bay. Her boyfriend Doug came to the service. He had forgotten what time we were supposed to meet to scatter Mom's ashes, he said.

Ken brought a Bible and led us in prayers. Angie, who accompanied me when I met my mother those few times, gave the euology, ending with, "I'd like to share a profound thought on life and death, recorded from Apollonius of Tanya in the first century A.D.:

"There is no death of anything save in appearance. That which passes over from essence to nature seems to be birth, and what passes over from nature to essence seems to be death. Nothing really is originated, and other ever perishes, but only now comes into sight and now vanishes."

And then she said, "And as all is connected in the universe, James and his mother and all who have connected in love remain unified in love forever and ever."

I went home early, lay down on my bed and curled up in a ball. Hours passed. It was the blackest I had ever felt. With Mom gone, I couldn't believe I had anything left to live for.

The titles of my favorite Pink Floyd albums echoed around in my head. *The dark side of the moon. Wish you were here. Eclipse. Speak to me. Comfortably numb.*

A staff psychologist came and sat by me, explaining that it was perfectly normal to feel so empty. I shouldn't be afraid to let it out.

Time passed, we ate and did dishes. I went to work, put together packets and answered the phone. Went to the mall, talked to people, got admitted to the hospital, got out of the hospital.

For years I just went through the motions of living, trying to remember why I was supposed to like living. I knew I was supposed to feel grateful that I was surrounded by helping hands, but I didn't feel much at all. I was just letting grief out.

But while I was letting grief out, although I didn't realize it, I was also starting to let something in.

Chapter 16

BEHIND THE DAY PROGRAM FACILITIES AND
the offices of West Bay Residential Services is a river bank
shaded by trees. The slow river meanders past so quietly
on its path to Narragansett Bay and the Atlantic, people
often forget it is there.

During spring of 2010, Rhode Island received 20.15
inches of rain in 38 days. The soil was as saturated as a
wet paper towel. When heavy rains began again in late
March, all the water of that downpour rolled directly
into already-engorged rivers, streams and reservoirs. The
Pawtuxet River crested at nearly 21 feet, more than 11
feet above flood stage.

On Tuesday, March 30, I was just settling in to a long
day of work when I received a phone call from home.

"We'll be there to pick you up in a few minutes," said
the team member on duty. The bus that had dropped

me off wouldn't be able to get to me quickly enough to rescue me, he said.

While I was still on the phone, Vivian, our human resources director, came rushing in to tell me that everyone was leaving early. "It's getting really bad out there, and Ted wants to make sure everyone is safe."

When Marta from my house showed up, she drove to a nearby Subway to grab sandwiches. We weren't usually at home for lunch and there was nothing there for us to eat. A river was growing in the parking lot. We got out of there before it became impassable, and barely made it home before the street in front of our house turned into a lake.

It was the worst flooding in over 200 years for the area, swamping the Warwick Mall, and many homes in the area, forcing many evacuations across Rhode Island and Southeastern Massachusetts. The flooding also caused many schools to close for an extended period of time, due to road impassability and washouts. The river crept into the offices of West Bay Residential services and destroyed nearly everything.

Perhaps worst of all, because sewage treatment plants failed, the water supply was contaminated.

"Don't drink unboiled water. Don't wash your clothes. Don't take showers," government officials warned us through local news broadcasters.

For four days we lived as if under siege by terrorists. It reminded me of September 11, 2001, and all my dark thoughts about the precariousness, the injustice, and the futility of life resurfaced.

September 11 is my birthday. Sometimes it's really hard not to give in to the temption to believe that everything about me and my life is unlucky.

After the flood, came the rebuilding. Cleanup took a month, and then the building was safe enough for me to go back to work, stuffing the day packets we needed to keep at least a few programs running smoothly. I was working in the offices, in the middle of a construction zone for a couple of months before all of our programs were up and running.

This is what survivors do. After the flood washes away the life we had, with the help and by the grace of God, we go back to work and we make a new life.

Natural disasters, especially when they come in the midst of a major recession, are costly. Money for programming became tight, and we needed to figure out inexpensive ways to spend our leisure time.

Writing poetry had brought me peace and pleasure, so I suggested we write poetry as a group. Sara, our day program director at the time thought it was a good idea.

So every week on Thursdays at 2:00, we would gather as a group to write poems. We didn't really know what we were doing, but we were having fun, listening to each other and sharing our thoughts and feelings.

The poetry group brought people together and built a sense of trust. The book *Thursdays at 2: poems to gladden the heart* tells that story, so I won't retell it here.

(Yeah, that was a clever ploy to get you to buy our poetry book, the sales of which help support creative ventures for individuals served by West Bay Residential Services--it's available on Amazon. Also, it will teach you how to use poetry to foster deeper, more meaningful connections in your own group.)

What happened for me is that through the process of writing poems with the people who surround my life today, I changed my attitude about the past.

For a long time I thought all those years spent trying to connect with my mom and trying to make her love me, had been a failure and a waste of time. But they weren't a waste. They were a journey I took, and that's where I learned an important truth about relationships.

When I'm looking for love and acceptance, it doesn't work to chase after the people who have failed me, rejected me, or left this earth. If I want to be loved, I have to open my heart to the people who are right here with me, right now. I have to take them into my heart so that we can share love and acceptance with each other.

In order to do that, I had to learn not to hold everyone else responsible for my own happiness or misery. That took some time, and I needed a lot of help. The big battle isn't with everyone out there, with my housemates, coworkers, with the government, or with the ignorant people who think that I'm not quite human because I'm in a wheelchair.

The real battle is against the dark side of my personality. I don't want to be mistrustful, cynical, feeling like a victim. I don't want to assume that because I have a disability, everyone ought to treat me well even if I verbally attack them. I want to be the kind of person who supports other people in hard times. I want to be like the people who have helped me grow.

But the reality is, I live in a frail, disabled body, weakened by a birth defect and multiple illnesses, and unable to walk. It took a lot of growing up before I realized how futile it is to chase after deluded dreams in which I become a teacher or famous writer and rescue my mom from the consequences of her choices. Life goes better when I accept the life, and the limitations, I have been given.

Accepting and forgiving my mother, accepting and forgiving my own weaknesses, and and accepting and forgiving everyone who doesn't give me what I think I ought to have—those are the first three steps toward a good life. And the next step is to take responsibility for doing the work that will make my life better.

My family taught me that.

For most of my life, I thought my family was made up of the people who are related to me by blood. But now I understand that the people who are willing to commit to a relationship with me, who will stand by me when life is hard, and celebrate with me when things go well—those people are my real family.

And this is how I live now—day by day, without my mother, with spina bifida, in the company of the amazing, faithful people who have taught me to dare to believe that I matter to them as much as they matter to me.

Thank you, my people. You know who you are.

About the Author

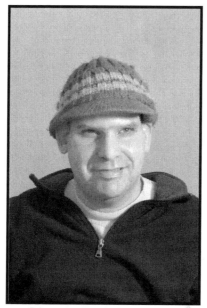

Photo by Rachel McKenna

James Boucher was a past member of the West Bay Residential Services Board of Directors, and holds a job as an administrative assistant, collating day activities packets for all of the group homes supported by West Bay. James is also the man who came up with the idea of making collaborative poetry at West Bay. In 1996 he was awarded the Ginsberg Prize for his poem, *I Put Pen to Paper*.

From 2010 to 2015, he collaborated with the West Bay Poets to produce the volume *Thursdays at 2: poems to gladden the heart*.

67695514R00051

Made in the USA
San Bernardino, CA
25 January 2018